*The International Library o_*

PLEASURE AND PAIN

Founded by C. K. Ogden

The International Library of Psychology

PHYSIOLOGICAL PSYCHOLOGY
In 10 Volumes

PLEASURE AND PAIN

A Theory of the Energic Foundation of Feeling

PAUL BOUSFIELD

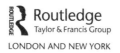
Routledge
Taylor & Francis Group

LONDON AND NEW YORK

First published in 1926
by Routledge, Trench, Trubner & Co., Ltd.
2 Park Square, Milton Park, Abingdon, Oxfordshire OX14 4RN
711 Third Avenue, New York, NY 10017

First issued in paperback 2014

Routledge is an imprint of the Taylor and Francis Group, an informa business

British Library Cataloguing in Publication Data
A CIP catalogue record for this book
is available from the British Library

Pleasure and Pain
ISBN 0415-21073-9
Physiological Psychology: 10 Volumes
ISBN 0415-21131-X
The International Library of Psychology: 204 Volumes
ISBN 0415-19132-7

ISBN 13: 978-1-138-88256-0 (pbk)
ISBN 13: 978-0-415-21073-7 (hbk)

CONTENTS

v

PAGE

CONTENTS

PREFACE

THE theory contained in the following pages embodies some lectures given by the author in 1923, and is the result of an attempt to treat the tension aspect of pleasure and pain not as a symbolic expression, but as a fact, and one which has quite probably an important part to play in the theory of feeling, and perhaps of consciousness itself. I have sought to demonstrate the nature of the relation I see between the various factors present in the feeling-processes by means of a series of diagrams which are, however, ideal representations and not exact ones, and in doing so I have confined myself deliberately to a fairly obvious set of examples.

An element of tension is generally recognised as present in states of feeling, though it does not receive very much consideration so far as I am aware. Yet states of tension appear to be the fundamental condition underlying all phenomena, whether in the organic or the inorganic world. Any factor which appears to be common to organic and inorganic substance, and, perhaps, even to consciousness itself, is worth investigating ; though for that very reason it will require investigating with the greater care. The nature of psychic tension is unknown.

The hypothesis of which this work is but a part can have many applications, but the author has touched here briefly upon two of them only, viz., instinct and the Freudian libido theory. The consideration of the tension does not solve the problem of the nature of the processes studied, but perhaps helps to state the problem in a form in which it may admit of being carried further.

I desire to express my thanks to Mr. W. R. Bousfield, K.C., F.R.S., and Miss R. Easterling, M.A., for reading my manuscript and giving me many valuable suggestions as to the form this short work should take. I also wish to take this opportunity of thanking Dr. W. M. Clement for preparing the diagrams and reading the proofs, and Miss M. B. Waller, B.Sc., for permission to include certain diagrams from the researches of her father, the late Prof. Waller, F.R.S.

PAUL BOUSFIELD.

October, 1925.
  7 Harley Street,
        London.

PLEASURE AND PAIN

PART I

Tension, Pleasure, and Pain.

Psychology has produced various theories concerning the nature of pain and pleasure and the inter-relation of the two. In particular, the pleasure of enjoying pain, as in masochism, has presented serious difficulties. Attempts to trace the source of masochism have been made by means of analytical methods, but the difficulty which has always arisen in such analytical procedure has been that the memories of the subject could never be taken far enough back into childhood, and thus the ultimate causes remained largely speculative. I was fortunate enough to be able to collect some new data from observations on a case in which the subject remembered a series of stages in the formation of a masochistic temperament, which I shall refer to further in a later part of this thesis.

The problem of masochism occupied my attention primarily, but it led to the formation of a working hypothesis of the foundation of pleasure and pain, which is here put forward.

It will be seen that I have approached the matter from the point of view of negative or unpleasant feeling-tone rather than the positive or pleasant aspect, and I have taken for illustration the phenomena arising in connection with such sensations as hunger and thirst, which have the advantage of enabling us to make readier use of certain biological conceptions.

But since the nature of the problem I started with was a psychic one, *viz.*, the feeling aspect of a very complex mental disposition (masochism), I had also to make use of the light thrown on the problem by various psychic states which have undeniably unpleasant feeling-tone. It appears, however, that the feeling-tone of the more complicated emotional structures with which the analyst deals will often be found to range itself, through association of ideas, with that of much more elementary states of feeling.

The hypothesis I formed has the advantage that it can be applied, not only to masochism or so-called enjoyment of pain, but to other problems that present themselves as well.

In this work I frequently use the terms

pleasure and pain in the sense of pleasant and unpleasant affect, and the term pain may include both sensation and affect, for a distinction at this point does not seem to affect my hypothesis. Moreover, as will be seen, pain is no true antithesis of pleasure. I do not believe that those who are familiar with the results of mental analysis will object to the term *painful* as applied to the affect of various mental and psychic conditions, and I, therefore, have no hesitation in using such expressions as " pain-curve " and " tension manifested in consciousness as pain."

Freud* and other writers tell us that pain and pleasure are related to the quantity of excitation present in the psychic life, and I might also mention the theory of Ziehen, that it is the *dischargability* of nervous excitation that determines the feeling-process.†
He says : " The affections have . . . to do with . . . excitation itself and its dischargability . . . . The positive feeling processes correspond to a greater readiness for discharge, the negative feeling processes to a smaller readiness."

* S. Freud, *Beyond the Pleasure Principle*, p. 2.

† Ziehen, *Physiologische Psychologie der Gefühl und Affekte*, cited by Wohlgemuth, *British Journal of Psychology*, 1917, p. 466.

But we shall have to go further than this, and that is why I wish to consider especially the tension aspect of these states. The difficulty of tracing causes far enough back by means of psychological analysis, determined me to begin at the other end of the argument, and to see if observations in biology, and deductions from physical phenomena, would lead to a point where the ground thus synthetically covered would meet with that previously explored by analysis.

Assuming that from the reactions of the lowest forms of life those of higher animals are developed, I commenced *de novo* with the question : What reactions are present in the lowest unicellular animals—that is to say, at a point in the scale of evolution at which neither consciousness nor feeling could be postulated ?   Could these reactions be described as instinctive ?   I had previously accepted, as axiomatic, at least two primitive instincts in the higher animals, *viz.*, the instinct for self-preservation and the instinct for the propagation of the species; both these tending in a broad sense to secure the continuity of life.

When the unicellular animals were regarded from the point of view of instinct, neither of

these so-called primordial instincts appeared
to be necessarily present. Stimuli and reactions to stimuli there were, and though
it is true that the reactions to stimuli tended
to preserve the species, there seemed to be no
evidence of any real instinct for such preservation. The same appeared to be the case
with propagation. As far as one could see,
fatigue, chemiotaxis, and other factors, led
to propagation, but definite instincts for such
could not be argued logically. In many cases
the same reactions to stimuli take place in
certain plants, yet we never speak of instincts
of either self-preservation or self-propagation
in plants. For instance, the propagation of
the spirogyra is closely allied to the propagation of the paramæcium, and the
fertilisation of ferns, in many instances, is
very similar to that of vertebrates.

"Instinct," in many ways, appears to
have been too readily accepted as an
explanation for various phenomena, which
are as easily explained by a mechanical
response to stimuli, frequently without any
" psychic " intervention at all. If we accept
as an instinct that phenomenon of " feigning
death," apparently used by many small
animals (certain spiders, etc., etc.), we shall

also accept as an instinct, exactly the same phenomenon when it occurs in plants. The *Mimosa Pudica*, for instance, is so sensitive to stimuli, that the disturbance caused by the footsteps of an approaching animal is sufficient to make all the leaves curl up and the branches droop. Heinrecker tells us that on entering a thick clump of bushes of the *Mimosa Pudica*, one is faced with a wall of tall, dense foliage, which, at each step taken, appears to recede before one, the original mass of rich vegetation transforming into an empty, burnt-out-looking space, enlarging with every forward stride. This appears to be protective, for it seems highly probable that the Mimosa avoids destruction of its leaves in a large degree by thus presenting an uninviting appearance to grazing animals ; moreover, many authorities have stated that neither oxen, horses, nor goats, will eat Mimosa. They sometimes attempt to do so, but the sudden movement and closing of its leaves appears to embarrass, if it does not frighten them. This is not an isolated instance. The wood sorrel closes its leaves at the slightest touch. The tendrils of the Passion Flower, and of the Trumpet Flower (*Bignonia*) behave similarly.

We may also cite the large variety of carnivorous plants which behave as though they possessed instinct. One of the most striking of these is the Venus Fly Trap, which has flat leaves hinged across the middle, with six sensitive bristles on the surface. As soon as the insect touches one of these the flower closes on it, marginal teeth lock the trap, and digestive juices absorb the insect. A near relative of this plant is the *Aldrovandia Vesiculosa* which, however, feeds not on flies, but on water-creatures. Compare these two plants with the sea anemone, which reacts to stimuli in exactly the same way.

It seems, on considering these facts, that we must regard the spider and other animals, not as "feigning death," but as reacting to certain stimuli purely in an automatic manner. That such a reaction leads to preservation of life is true, and "natural selection" tends to preserve those animals possessing forms of reaction to tension of this kind.

A similar explanation seems to hold good for many other so-called preservative "instincts."

Let us turn our attention, with these thoughts in mind, to animals higher in the

scale of evolution, and notice particularly
various experiments conducted by Dr Chalmers
Mitchell. All these experiments tended to
show that, in the majority of cases, there
appeared to be no knowledge of death nor of
hereditary enemies, nor any instinct of fear
in the animals observed, unless social heredity,
i.e., early education and experience had first
inculcated that fear.

Dr Chalmers Mitchell carried out experiments with young animals and snakes, since
the snake was supposed to be the most
terror-inspiring of all animals. He states that
every one of these species experimented on
showed "no special dread of snakes, nor the
slightest instinctive fear or fore-knowledge of
their approaching doom."* Of further experiments, he states :—

"Nearly every kind of mammal that we
tried was indifferent to snakes. Guinea-pigs
and rats would run over them ; a hyrax, which
is both intelligent and which, from living in
trees and on rocks, must often encounter
snakes, was hardly even interested. . . . .
Small carnivora—dogs, foxes, and wolves,
sheep, antelope and deer, zebras, and donkeys
—were either quite indifferent, or came up

* Dr Chalmers Mitchell, *The Childhood of Animals.*

to the bars and sniffed," and on finding that the snake was not something to eat, " moved away with an air of wearied disgust."

He also states that frogs, which are the natural food of snakes in this country, showed no fear, nor did most monkeys. A certain amount of fear was shown by the higher monkeys and by one or two of the more intelligent birds. But this, Dr Chalmers Mitchell considers to be not so much a case of inherited fear as an intellectual fear, caused by the unusual appearance and movement of the snake, which the more highly developed brain appreciated, but could not understand.

Other experiments carried out by Benjamin Kidd are also most conclusive. He states :*

" I experimented with a number of wild species of British birds and mammals. In none of them did I find any trace in the young of an inborn, instinctive fear of the natural enemies which were regarded with fear and terror by the adult of the species. Young wild hares and young wild rabbits showed no inborn fear of either cats or dogs. Young wild rabbits and young wild hares became as friendly and playful from the beginning with specially trained cats to which they were

* Benjamin Kidd, *The Science of Power.*

introduced, as if they had been all of the same
species. Young rabbits showing no inborn
fear of dogs, would frisk and play with the
hereditary enemy of their kind, by whom their
species had been hunted for tens of thousands
of generations. The young of our common
wild birds showed no inborn fear of the cat
when, fully fledged, they were, under proper
conditions, introduced to it for the first time.
Nor did they develop any fear afterwards.
And so also when they were introduced under
similar conditions to birds of prey like the
hawk, or the carrion crow, trained to friendly
relations.

"If it be asked now, whence comes the
universal and ineradicable fear of natural
enemies, which is present under natural
conditions in the whole of the adult members
of the species in these cases, the answer is of
great interest. *The conclusion which I arrived
at was that in the numerous typical wild
species experimented upon, the whole of this
powerful influence, representing a most dominant
and ineradicable habit of animal nature, was
entirely the result of social heredity imposed on
the young of each generation by training and
example, and nearly always under conditions
of strong emotion. . . .* The record of a single

example will exhibit the meaning that was found to be inherent in a great number of experiments. I came on a nest of the wild duck in a marsh as the young birds had just emerged from the eggs. The mother duck flew off and disappeared in the sedge, flapping a wing to which she pretended injury. I stood by the nest for some hours and watched the young birds. The greatest number were already active and displaying an interest in their surroundings. They began to try and get out of the nest, and I took them one by one in my hand and placed them in the water, where, in the stillness that reigned, they splashed and twittered and enjoyed themselves. They showed not the slightest fear of me, nestling from time to time on my feet, and turning intelligent eyes upwards to look at me, evidently quite ready to accept me in the fullest confidence as their guardian.

" The wild duck had been in these marshes for untold ages. She had been here even in the days when the woolly rhinoceros left its remains with those of the cavemen in the adjacent hills. During all this time her kind had been one of the most universally hunted among wild creatures. The spent cartridges of the modern sportsman strewed the bog around, yet here were her off-spring just entering on the world and showing no sign of any kind of inborn fear of this, the hereditary enemy of the species.

" After a time I moved away some distance to watch what would happen. The mother bird returned and alighted near by. The little ducks rushed towards her as she called. I could observe her. She was chattering with emotion. Every feather was quivering with excitement. The great Terror of Man was upon her. After a short interval I advanced towards the group again. The mother bird flew away with a series of loud warning quacks. The little ones scattered to cover, flapping their short wing stumps and cheeping with beaks wide open in terror. With difficulty I found one of them again in hiding. It was now a wild, transformed creature, trembling in panic which could not be subdued.

" It is in this way, and under conditions of the strongest emotion, that the accumulated experience of tens of thousands of generations of the species is imposed on young birds. Once having received it, within a few days, even within a few hours, they pass into another world, from which they can never be reclaimed."

It will be noticed that in the higher monkeys and the more intelligent birds, a certain amount of fear was exhibited, and Dr. Chalmers Mitchell suggests that this was due to the higher imagination of these animals, by means of which anything strange would instil fear. When we are afraid, it is because the imagination presents something to us. It is not necessarily an instinct of fear so much as a reasoned fear, based on the experience that strange things are the possible causes of pain.

From the evidence here quoted, it appeared obvious that if there were an instinct of self-preservation in the animals mentioned, it acted in a remarkably poor manner as an instinct. Therefore, one sought another solution for the cause of the activities observed in wild animals, which, in effect, does preserve their lives. One realised that in the higher animals, the instinct or desire to avoid pain would be equally efficacious, for the process of being killed from without, or poisoned from within, is generally accompanied by pain, and since pain in one form or another is felt by all animals possessing consciousness from birth onwards, and probably also during the act of birth, their experience would very soon tend to make them avoid all occasions where pain might be expected to supervene. Whereas, if consciousness and imagination had not been developed, or were of an extremely low order, they would not be afraid, and strange objects would convey to them no idea of pain, especially if such objects had considerable resemblance to other objects which did not cause pain. Thus, a snake is not unlike the roots of a tree, except that it moves, it is not unlike a worm, it is not unlike the creepers and branches which animals are used to seeing in their native life; indeed, by its very similarity to these things, it is enabled to obtain its prey and a tame animal, which has never seen a snake, and need, therefore, fear no pain from it because it has not been educated on that subject by the parent animal, would be unlikely to fear it.

When one advances this idea further into the domain of human imagination, one may say that the recoil from death, which most of us seem to possess, by no means necessarily represents an instinct of self-preservation, but represents a fear of something painful and exists on account of two reasons. The first of these is that death is associated with accident, illness and pain, and the second is that there is frequently a fear induced by

the imagination of an unknown hereafter.
Later on we shall, I think, discover a third
and very potent reason for avoiding death.
There are tribes in whom the fear of death
appears to be almost absent, and this is
probably because they are so certain of the
type of hereafter which will be experienced,
that they have no fears concerning it, and
their early environment has weakened the
other factor, to which I shall refer later.
However this may be, the conclusion I came
to was, that we certainly had no evidence for
asserting that such an instinct as the instinct
of self-preservation really existed. We had,
however, considerable evidence, and know that
an "instinct" for the avoidance of pain or,
as we shall see later, an avoidance of tension,
does exist. That a true instinct of self-
preservation does not exist is further suggested
by other observations of Dr Chalmers Mitchell,
if the deductions he makes are right, for he
states that he does not consider that young
animals have any instinct for avoiding
poisonous food, as has so frequently been
heretofore assumed.*

* Dr Chalmers Mitchell, *Op. cit.*, p. 244.

§2

Let us now return to our unicellular animal, or to our sensitive plant, or to such other forms of life as apparently have no brain and no nervous system such as we know it, and, therefore, we are inclined to assume, possess no consciousness and no imagination, and, therefore, no actual sensation of pain as such. We must ask ourselves, of what, then, does this pain consist, and how is it that these living things without pain still continue to preserve themselves ? The reply, of course, is that they react automatically to certain stimuli. We may go back to our amœba and see how it reacts to stimuli. First, however, let us remember what is the universal result of any stimulus—whether in the organic or inorganic world. It may be described as a state of tension.

We see this state of tension marked in the amœba by a certain amount of contraction at the point of tension. For instance, if a grain of cochineal or of suitable food be placed so that the amœba comes against it in the course of its progression, the point at which

contact is established tends slightly to con-
tract, and ceases for the moment to move
forward, while so-called pseudo-podia are
thrown forward to engulf the morsel. The
animalcule continues to move forward at
points on either side of the morsel, which has
caused the stimulus, and which in turn has
resulted in that portion in the immediate
neighbourhood of the stimulus remaining
stationary. In other words, the feeding of
the amœba is very much like the flowing of
water round a rock which is placed in its path.
The immediate result of a minute particle
coming in contact with the amœba is to cause
the immediate neighbourhood of the point of
contact to become stationary. A stimulus
applied to the whole body of the amœba, such
as an unsuitable fluid, causes this reaction at
all points, and the amœba contracts into a
circular form. A similar reaction takes place
whether food is presented or whether a merely
mechanical stimulus of indigestible dust is
given to it. Apparently any stimulus results
in contraction of the stimulated part, or, as
we may put it, *in a state of tension* of the
stimulated part. When the particle has
been engulfed by the amœba, the tension
causes a flow of the digestive fluid, and if the

particle be digestible, it is absorbed, or partially absorbed.   If it be wholly absorbed, the
state of tension is got rid of in this way.   If
it be partially absorbed, the vacuole in which
it rests continues to be irritated until the
amount of fluid which is secreted bursts it,
and the indigestible material is expelled,
so that in either case the state of tension is
relieved, either by digestion or by such an
increase of fluid as may cause disruption.

But in all this, let us note in passing, we
see no signs of a so-called instinct of self-
preservation.   Likewise, we do not see any
instinct of reproduction so far as we can
tell.   When metabolism or the products of
metabolism in the protoplasm of the animalcule has caused a given condition of internal
stimulation, a state of tension is produced
which leads to activity of the nucleus, and to
reproduction by mere fission of the animal.

If we transfer these ideas to animals which
are higher in the scale, we see a similar state
of affairs in existence.   Let us take hunger
in the human being.   When no meal has been
eaten for several hours certain specialized
contractions (and probably other stimuli)
are present in increasing force, together with
certain psychic stimuli.   The latter we shall

for the moment neglect since we shall introduce the subject of psychic reflexes and
imagination shortly. These stimuli cause a
state of local irritation. They produce a
condition of tension in the nerve endings,
which is accompanied by a state of psychic
tension in consciousness, which we call hunger,
and hunger belongs undeniably to the category
of pain, *i.e.*, it has unpleasant feeling tone.
When food is taken the stimuli are neutralised
and hence the tension is removed, and we
associate the relief of this tension, that is the
eating of food, with pleasure. If we consider
this, and simultaneously bear in mind the
working of the amœba, it is forced on our
attention that stimuli tend to cause pain when
consciousness is present, and that the removal
of tension causes pleasure. The immediate
result of these stimuli, when the nervous
system is sufficiently developed and consciousness has become present, has been the consciousness of pain. The question then arises,
do all stimuli cause pain ? Or are there such
things as pleasurable stimuli *per se* ? This, at
the present juncture, we will not assume. We
can think of a number of stimuli which cause
instant contraction and tension, as did the
particle in contact with the amœba. An

extreme instance in our own case would be contact with the surface of the cornea, which is furnished with pain nerves. What is meant, however, by saying that stimuli of themselves tend to cause tension will be realised by anyone who watches a spirited horse or dog quivering with sensitive movement in every part, in response to all the slight sounds and other stimuli of its surroundings.

We see no immediate need to think that there are such things as pleasurable stimuli. The suggestion comes to us that pleasure may only be the result of the removal of tension or pain. If we look once more at our amœba, at our sensitive plant, or at any living organism which does not possess a definite nervous system, this idea seems to hold perfectly good throughout. We see a series of activities regularly taking place, stimuli causing states of tension, and the state of tension then being relieved, and a state of non-tension, or reduced tension again produced. And we may even formulate a law that *every substance in a state of tension tends to reduce that tension.* But when we come to the realm of human beings, the matter seems to be by no means as clear.

At first sight, there appear to be many pleasurable and many neutral stimuli, but if we

examine them we shall find in the less complicated forms of pleasure that this is not of
necessity the case, for a new factor has been
introduced, which of its own account can
produce both tension and relief of tension
apart from physical stimuli. This is the
imagination (acting, of course, only in the
presence of consciousness) which produces
direct psychic or mental stimuli without the
intervention of physical stimuli, and causes a
state of psychic tension which it can also
discharge. There is another important factor
to be reckoned with : that there is always a
pre-existing state of tension in the organism,
the condition of its very existence in relation
to its environment, but this I shall refer to
more fully later on, and will content myself
here with one example of it. Whilst it must
be admitted that we enjoy drinking when we
are thirsty and obtain pleasure as a result
of the removal of the unpleasant state of
tension manifested in consciousness as thirst,
there are many people who apparently enjoy
drinking when they are not thirsty, and it
would seem on the face of it, as though the
·fluid itself, or the flavour thereof, caused a
pleasurable stimulus. But I think that a
series of observations will convince us that

C

this is not the case. An analysis of any one who is inclined towards alcohol, for instance, whether in a large or small quantity, will show that the alcohol is taken to relieve some already existing state of tension.

There are some complicated issues connected with this class of stimuli, with flavours and with food, as well as with other different kinds of stimuli, which I do not propose to enter into at present, for I wish to cover some of the simpler ground first.

§3

Let us now examine in a little more detail the part played by imagination as a tension producer and reliever.

It is well known that within certain limits the greater the hunger or thirst the greater the pleasure we have in relieving it. But there are times when the pleasure of relieving the tension may be present before the actual relief takes place. It is by no means uncommon, for instance, to hear a man remark that he has a " glorious thirst." We have most of us known, after a long and hot ramble in the country, the pleasurable anticipation as the goal came in sight where we could relieve our thirst. The tension of thirst is still present, yet there is also pleasure present, but that pleasure is present because we have begun already to reduce that tension in consciousness, by means of our imagination.

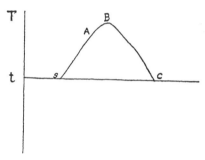

FIG. 1.

Pain and pleasure can, of course, exist only in consciousness.

Let me try to represent what happens in various cases by means of a few diagrams.   In these diagrams "T" represents the amount of tension produced, "t" represents the time during which it is acting.   Let us take first the case of an amœba.   A sudden stimulus, such as contact with a solid digestible particle, is produced at S (fig. 1) and an almost immediate rise to a full state of tension would probably take place, represented by part of the curve, S—A. The particle is then engulfed, and the tension remains nearly stationary or slowly rising for a short time ; this period is represented by A—B.

This particle would then begin to be slowly absorbed, and as the absorption takes place, the tension would probably be removed gradually, as represented by the line B—C and at the point C the tension has disappeared with complete digestion of the particle.

Let us now examine a simple example on the same lines, but in an animal possessing consciousness, taking for example the question of hunger. Again there is a gradual increasing tension in the cells of the stomach. This condition is conveyed *via* the nerves to the brain cells, and it sets up a corresponding tension of a psychic nature, which is manifested in consciousness by the unpleasant sensation of hunger and referred back to the stimulated physical cells. It does not much matter whether we plot our curve as physical tension or psychic tension, for the latter is dependent on the former, and appears under normal circumstances to be proportional to it. We shall. therefore. deal with the tension as

produced in the brain rather than that produced locally in the gastric cells, as this will
simplify our later comparisons. In fig. 2
then, we shall represent an individual who
has had no food for some time and whose
tension, due to various gastric stimuli is

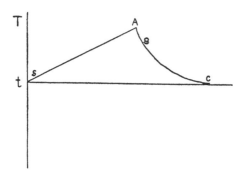

FIG. 2.

rising.   This rise of tension is once more
represented by the part of the curve S—A.
At the point A, food is taken, and the tension
is immediately reduced ; this reduction of
tension is shown by the part of the curve
A—B—C. If we take our awareness of the
sensation of hunger as representing the degree
of tension present, it will readily be realised,
both from introspection and analogy, that
the rate of relief of tension is much more

rapid during the first few mouthfuls, from A to B, than when the subject is approaching repletion at C—hence the concave shape of our curve.

Let us now introduce the question of feeling-tone. In fig. 1, since there was no consciousness we postulate no pain and no pleasure (pleasant or unpleasant affect). There is simply a state of tension and relief of tension, and at that we must leave it. But in fig. 2 our curve does not merely represent physical tension, but the mental equivalent of physical tension, which we may call psychic tension, and which is represented in consciousness by sensations and feeling tone. Let us see how this unpleasant affect corresponds with the tension. It would appear that the degree of unpleasant affect is relatively proportional to the degree of tension present. This idea is substantiated by consideration of other forms of painful tension. That of thirst appears to be proportional to the tension produced ; the painful affect under pressure such as pinching, is relatively proportional to the pressure-stimulus and hence to the tension. Whatever factors appear to increase the tension, also appear to add to the discomfort. The rate at which the various tensions are produced seems to have but little bearing on the degree of pain present. Thus we may get as thirsty in a very dry, hot atmosphere in the course of an hour as we should in a more humid atmosphere in the course of three hours. Experiences of various kinds lead us to the conclusion that, speaking generally, the pain (displeasure) experienced under any condition, is relatively proportional to the actual tension present, and has no relation to the time taken to produce that tension. Subject, therefore, to such modifications as may be represented by the difference in sensitivity of different cells, or the degree of consciousness present, we may say that pain is proportional to tension. We may elaborate it slightly by writing it as

$$P=T.S.C.$$

where P=pain, T=tension, and S and C represent constants of sensitivity and consciousness respectively. For elementary purposes we may, therefore, represent the pain curve representing displeasurable feeling as being the same as the tension curve from the point S to the point A (fig. 2).

When we come to examine the pleasure produced by the relief of tension, however,

the same does not hold good. For we observe
in hunger and thirst that the greatest pleasure
is produced with the first few mouthfuls, *i.e.*,
while the tension is still high and hunger
and thirst are still present, and as the tension
falls nearer to zero so does this pleasure
disappear. Moreover, we find that pain and
pleasure are at the highest point present
simultaneously—*i.e.*, hunger and enjoyment
of eating. And in this instance we first
observe that pain and pleasure are not anti-
thetical. If we consider the two examples
given above, and other examples to be mentioned later, we see that pleasure appears to
be in some measure proportional to the rate
of *fall* of tension ; thus, if we were thirsty,
we should get but little pleasure from the
relief effected by injecting water, drop by
drop, over a period of an hour—although at
the end of that time the tension and thirst
would have disappeared just as effectively
as they do by taking a large draught of water.
The same feature may be found in the relief
of other forms of tension, *i.e.*, the greatest
pleasure appears to be felt at the point of
maximum rate of fall of tension.

It is clear then that in the simple examples
taken, we cannot legitimately express pain

and pleasure in the same curve, for they are functions of different types of factor. If we were to compare them with dynamic factors, we might say that pain resembled a function of velocity, while pleasure represented a function of rate of change of velocity in an opposite direction. Since pleasure (in these simple examples) is thus a factor of time, as well as of tension, we may represent it by the formula :—

$$\pi = \frac{dT}{dt} \, S.C.$$

or

$$\pi = Tan \; \theta \; S.C.$$

where π represents the amount of pleasure, and S and C represent the constants of sensitivity and consciousness. We shall, therefore, have to project another curve from the curve A—C, according to this formula, in order to represent our pleasure. This we shall proceed to do in fig. 3, and for the moment we shall neglect the factors S and C.

In fig. 3 we depict a gradual rise of tension from S to A. At A a sudden fall takes place. This fall is represented from A to B by a drop of 10 in 1, from B to C by a drop of 10 in 3, from C to D by a drop of 10 in 6,

from D to E by a drop of 6 in 10, from E
to F. by a drop of 3 in 10, and so on.

Let us now plot the pain and pleasure curves
from this. As already stated, the pain curve
is efficently registered by the formula P=T,
i.e., by the line S A. The pleasure curve,
represented by $\pi = \frac{dT}{dt}$, is plotted below, thus :

From A to B $\frac{dT}{dt} = 10$ and is shown at a

„   B to C $\frac{dT}{dt} = \frac{10}{3} = 3.3$ „   „   „   „ b

„   C to D $\frac{dT}{dt} = \frac{10}{6} = 1.6$ „   „   „   „ c

„   D to E $\frac{dT}{dt} = \frac{6}{10} = .6$ „   „   „   „ d

„   E to F $\frac{dT}{dt} = \frac{3}{10} = .3$ „   „   „   „ e

Thus a—b—c—d—e, represents our pleasure
curve, and we at once observe that pleasure
is not proportional in any way to the amount
of tension (or of pain) present *per se*, and that
with even a small amount of tension, a great
amount of pleasure can be obtained if we
can make the rate of fall sufficiently rapid.
This is again borne out by introspectively
examining our experiences. Moderate thirst,
or hunger, may give us as much pleasure in
our food as extreme thirst or extreme hunger.

The sudden complete cessation of a mild headache, or toothache, gives as much pleasure as the sudden reduction of a severe pain of a similar kind to a moderate pain. In both cases the pleasure is evanescent, and in the second case we are very soon conscious of

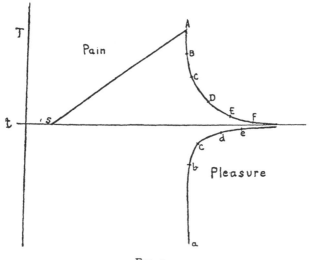

FIG. 3.

pain only—when no more reduction of tension is taking place. We shall, however, see these various ideas supported more conclusively by other examples as we proceed. We have already observed the converse that where tension falls very slowly, little pleasure is experienced, *i.e.*, in the relief of thirst by drops of water ; or we might cite the case of damaged or bruised tissues, which recover very slowly.

It must not, however, be taken that this simple formula, as it stands,

$$\pi = \frac{dT}{dt} \text{ s.c.}$$

is intended to represent any exact measure of pleasure. It simply represents the general type of curve which we might expect in simple cases, and it may be modified by many other constants. For instance, if " t " is infinitely small, we do not get infinite pleasure ; there is a limit to both pleasure and pain, which is not expressed in either the pain or pleasure formula.

§4

But there is another factor which we must introduce, which displaces these curves, as it were. So far, we have been treating the normal animal as though it completely lacked tension during part of its life, and, as though the effort were to get back to a state of relaxation, but even the amœba must be continually in some state of tension, and when we turn our attention to the higher animals, this becomes more obvious. Tension, it is known, is a fundamental condition of all being, organic and inorganic. With the human being the time of least tension (but not of complete absence of tension), is in the first three or four months of the intra-uterine life, when an even temperature is maintained, when there is no hunger, for a continual state of feeding, *via* the blood-stream, is taking place, when no efforts of respiration are required, and no struggle for life exists. As soon, however, as the fœtus begins to move, tension of some sort is produced, and at birth a series of efforts have to be made to live and breathe. Continual stimuli are entailed herewith : the stimuli of the respiratory centre of the brain (*i.e.*, the tension caused by the hydrogen-ion concentration of the blood), the stimuli of hunger, and so forth ; and, as is well known, the child often resents these mild stimuli and desires most to fall back into the condition simulating the intra-uterine condition as nearly as possible—the effortless condition.

Thus we may take it that from the earliest

times, immediately after birth, there is certainly a very definite *normal* state of tension set up, which the infant tends to resent. And although it may adapt itself, in course of time, to this normal tension, there is probably always the unconscious desire to retire from it. We must, therefore, shift all our tension curves up, as it were, and in any future curves that we draw, we shall have to assume that there is always a certain positive tension, and that the tensions causing hunger and pain, etc., are super-imposed on the normal tension.

But let us remember that we are not usually conscious of this normal tension any more than we are conscious of the atmospheric pressure, and that efforts to relieve it must therefore be made largely unconsciously, or, at least, with the motive remaining un-conscious. However, for the moment, that does not concern us for we have dealt only with conscious results of physical tension, neglecting other factors, such as imagination, unconscious cerebration, or purely psychic functions. Therefore, let us re-cast our curve shown in fig. 3, by making allowance for the permanent normal physical tension to which we have just referred. In fig. 4 this is shown. X—S represents the steady normal tension of life due to various small stimuli, S—A represents the superimposed tension, due, in our familiar instance, to lack of food or water, and A—B—C—D—E, the discharge of hunger or thirst tension, which follows eating or drinking and leaves the

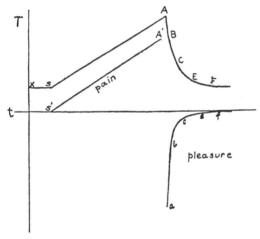

FIG 4.

subject in the normal state as before. But the normal tension does not exist in consciousness in the form of pain or displeasure, but is apparently neutral in tone, so that no corresponding shift must be made in the pain curve which will be represented by S'—A.' This will start at zero and come back to zero as

before. Nor will the pleasure curve be
changed if this depends on the rate of change
of tension. The importance of this modifi-
cation in our tension curve will be realised
later.

Let us summarise what we have so far been
considering :—

(1) Both the so-called instincts of self-
preservation and of reproduction appear
ultimately to be merely activities to relieve
tension caused by stimuli.

(2) In the case of self-preservation
the real instinct appears to be to avoid
the tension caused by *painful* stimuli
rather than the actual preservation of
life. (We have not considered this in
reference to reproduction).

(3) In these *simple cases* stimuli and states
of tension resulting therefrom cause pain
in animals which possess consciousness. Pain
appears, on the whole, to be generally proportional to tension, modified by certain
constants.

(4) In all similar cases pleasure appears
to be the result of relief from pain, *i.e.*, caused
by the neutralisation or discharge of tension
in animals which possess consciousness.
Pleasure appears, on the whole, to be generally

proportional to rate of change of tension, modified by certain constants.

§5

But let us now examine the effect of imagination. Now, imagination produces, though not exactly on the same scale nor exactly in the same way, a state of tension in many ways comparable with physical stimuli, whether internal or external, to the organism. It is as though the physical stimuli were imposed—yet they are not. As an example of this I may say that with Dr Waller, two or three years ago, I experimented with a hypnotised person. As those who have studied his experiments will know, painful stimuli altered the electrical resistance of the subject, which was measured by passing a continuous current through him and watching its effect on the galvanometer. If, for instance, a pin were suddenly stuck into the arm of the subject there would be a very definite alteration in his electrical resistance. And this could be shown in the form of curve, computed from the amplitude of movement of the galvanometer.

D

With my hypnotised subject, I found that
by merely touching his arm with a feather
and informing him that it was a pin, a similar
reaction was observed. Moreover, the same
occurred when I merely told him that a pin
was pricking him without the feather being
used as a physical stimulus. The mental
image of the pin-prick was enough without
the actual prick stimulus to produce the
physical reaction. And experiments by
Dr Waller, prior to this, had shown that even
in the normal individual the anticipation
of the pain of a pin prick would frequently
cause an even greater change of electrical
resistance in the subject than the prick itself.
Thus, if he allowed the subject to watch him
apparently about to jab the pin into his arm,
although at the last moment he did not
actually touch the subject, nevertheless the
psychic or emotional stimulus caused, in
many cases, an even greater change than the
prick itself, if it were applied without warning.
*On the whole, the nature of the electrical change
was much the same whether the stimulus were
of a physical or psychic nature.*
A large number of such experiments conclusively showed that stimuli produced by
the imagination were equivalent to physical

stimuli in the resulting tension produced.*
In every-day life we see similar psychic
stimuli at work. We know that the sight
of somebody sucking a lemon causes the flow
of saliva ; we know that the fear of a flogging
to come will cause a little boy to tremble and
cry—to react as though the flogging were
actually taking place, and although there
may be no actual feeling of physical pain, a
state of tension is produced in which there
is a mental reaction to pain as though it were
already there. We can, therefore, safely say
that a state of tension is produced in the
mind of the conscious animal by means of
imagination, and that this is in many ways
comparable to the state of tension produced
by the actual physical stimulus.

But just as a state of tension can be
produced in this way, so can a state of relief
be produced. We noticed earlier the mixed
case in which the thirsty man began to enjoy
the pleasure of drinking to relieve that thirst
when he came in sight of the relief, before he
actually relieved it. But let us try to examine
a case which is not mixed in this way : the
case of a child who sees some toy that it

* *Concerning Emotive Phenomena*, by A. D. Waller, M.D.,
F.R.S., in *Proceedings of the Royal Society*, B, Vol. 91, 1919.

desires and cries because it cannot possess it. A state of tension has been produced by the imagination of possessing the toy ; psychic pain is caused because the tension is present unreduced. If now somebody promises that to-morrow that toy shall be bought and given to the child, that state of tension is relieved.

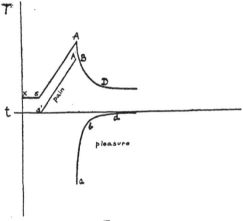

FIG. 5.

The child will cease crying and feel again a sense of pleasure, the whole situation being in this case a psychic one, and exactly the same curve as the last might be reproduced, the state of tension, owing to the desire to possess the toy, being represented by S—A (fig. 5), the feeling of psychic pain attached to it by S'—A', the reduction of the state of tension on the promise to fulfil the child's wish being represented by A—B—-D, this corresponding to a state of pleasure represented by a—b—d.

If at this point we want further evidence, not only of the similar states of tension caused by psychic and physical stimuli,

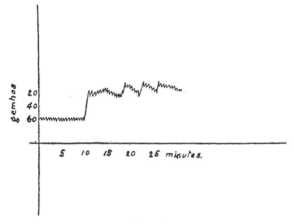

FIG. 6.

but also that the *tension appears to remain constant in proportion to the pain,* let us examine another of Dr Waller's* curves. Fig. 6 represents a curve taken during an air-raid on a certain individual. After the first interval of ten minutes there was the sound of

* Galvanometric records of the emotive response to air-raids, and to ordinary stimulation, real and imaginary.—*Lancet,* Feb. 23rd and Mar. 9th, 1918.

maroons, followed by that of aeroplanes and guns. The subject's resistance, which was previously about 60,000 ohms, fell at once to 20,000 ohms, and remained there during the 15 minutes depicted above. Here we are at once confronted with the continuous and level nature *of the tension caused by a continuous and definite psychic disturbance.*

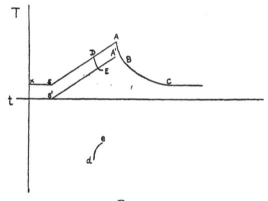

FIG. 7.

Now let us proceed to examine the case in which the psychic factor is superimposed on the physical one. Let us, as before, take the case of hunger or thirst: the physical tension actually present is accompanied by psychic tension, shown in fig. 7 by the rising curve S—A. At the point A, the tension begins to be relieved by actual food or drink and falls quickly along the portion A—B, and more gradually from B to C, at which point normal tension is again reached.

Simultaneously, there has been a beginning of pain at S', which would normally continue to A', but at the point D, the imagination of food or drink is introduced, and a relief of tension D—E in the psychic sphere takes place, causing a temporary appearance of pleasure, represented by d—e, so that pleasure actually begins, while pain is actually present, *i.e.*, while physical tension is still rising. We must, therefore, take it, and this is borne out by my actual experiments with the hypnotised subject that the imagination is able actually to inhibit psychic tension, due to physical tension under certain circumstances. But since, in the case quoted, the physical tension is still rising and hunger or thirst is still in consciousness, we must assume that the inhibition is only temporary and that, when it appears to be maintained, it is due to a series of rapid inhibitions alternating with periods during which the physical stimulus gains the upper hand and succeeds in reinstating the psychic tension represented by hunger or thirst.

Indeed, careful introspection assures us

that this is the case normally. For we observe that this pleasure obtained by the imagination under such circumstances is not continuous, and that we cannot, as a rule, hold our attention continuously on the anticipated relief.

The same idea is borne out in another experiment, quoted by Dr. Waller,* in which Miss G. de B. prepared an apparatus to take a 40 minute photographic record of her emotive state. She set herself the task of remaining emotionless during the first 20 minutes and emotionally unhappy during the next 20 minutes, which latter was secured by a voluntary recollection of air-raids, and of the "military execution" of a Belgian, witnessed at Termonde, in 1914. The record which is approximately reproduced (Fig. 8) shows that the imagination was unable to maintain complete control, and that a continual alteration of emotive response was taking place electrically during the effort.

Reverting now to the further consideration of the discharge of the tension during hunger or thirst by means of the imagination, we see that, although pleasure may be obtained by a series of rapid discharges of this tension, the

* *Op. cit.*

actual tension remains high and indeed continues to rise, so that unless the conscious
mind were so limited as to be completely
incapable of the realisation of two feelings at
once, we should (according to our formula
P=T) expect hunger to remain present in
consciousness, and this is actually the case.

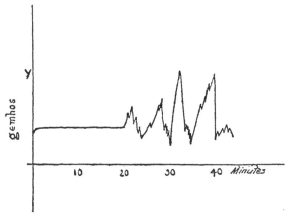

FIG. 8.

Whether the pleasure or the pain will predominate, will obviously depend on whether
T is greater or less than $\frac{dT}{dt}$ at any moment.
This, in turn, is to some extent dependent on
a " habit formation," as we shall see a little
later.   We shall, therefore, proceed to revise
our curve, shown in Fig. 7, in a new curve,
shown in Fig. 9.   In this we have represented

a series of tension discharges, due to the imagination at D, E, F, G, H, K, which are accompanied by pleasure impulses recorded at d, e, f, g, h, k. S′ to A′ represents as before, the increasing pain of hunger which is now, however, intermittent from D′ to A′—

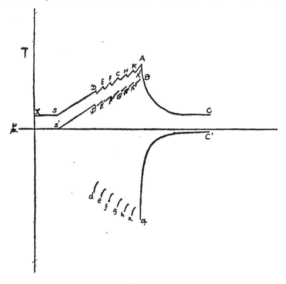

FIG. 9.

owing to alternating periods during which pleasure predominates. If, now, these alternations are sufficiently rapid, it would appear as if pain and pleasure were present simultaneously—which frequently does actually seem to be the case.

The psychic discharge of stimuli never gives complete relief of tension. Thus, as before stated, there appears to be both pain and pleasure present simultaneously, until the physical tension is relieved—at which point pleasure is enhanced. Thus we now distinguish two manifestations of pleasure; there is one due to physical relief, represented by the line a—c, which comes with the actual fall of physical tension, but there is another manifestation of pleasure, represented by lines d, e, f, g, etc., which we might call pseudo-pleasure, or, perhaps more intelligibly, *fore-pleasure. The latter can only . exist, however, in the normal course of events as long as the subject is aware that the point C will be ultimately reached.* If the hungry individual were suddenly informed that no refreshment were available at the place where he expected it, all fore-pleasure represented by d, e, f, g, etc., would disappear, while on the other hand, even were there no relief obtainable, so long as the subject imagined it possible, the tension discharge giving fore-pleasure would remain. This is important to remember, as we shall see at a later period, for we must now introduce another series of curves with an unconscious factor at work.

§6

As I stated at the beginning of this thesis,
I was fortunate in gaining a new series of
observations in one of my patients ; I was
also led to see the part played by unconscious
factors in this same subject.   I shall, therefore, at this stage, proceed to give some details
of the observations recorded.   I was fortunate,
in the case I am about to relate, in being able
to elicit the history of a continued change
gradually taking place.   The case was that
of a patient who had gradually substituted
fore-pleasure for end-pleasure in a large
number of spheres of activity.   That is to say,
he substituted psychic discharges for physical
discharges of tension, and in order to lengthen
his period of psychic fore-pleasure, he postponed the discharge of physical tension by
deliberately adding stimuli to protract the
tension indefinitely.

One of his earliest recollections as a small
boy was of throwing off the bedclothes so that
he got very cold, and lying in this state for a
few minutes ; he then put on the bedclothes
again.   He did this in order to obtain the

great pleasure of feeling warm once more.
He was willing to undergo the painful stimulus
in order to obtain the pleasure at the end.
The tension curve in this instance is represented in fig. 10 by the line S—A.   At A the

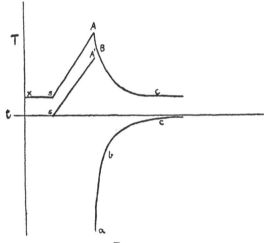

Fig. 10.

bedclothes were put on again, and the tension
rapidly reduced as represented by A—B—C.
Corresponding with this curve is the pain
curve S'—A', and the projected pleasure
curve, a—b—c.   Gradually a change took
place in his method, it is represented
in fig. 11.   The bedclothes, as before, were
thrown off at the point marked S.   The
maximum tension due to cold was reached

at A, and then continued, perhaps, for an hour or more. At the point B the bedclothes were put on again, and the reduction of tension is shown by B—C. In this instance the maximum of physical pain was reached at A', which corresponds with the

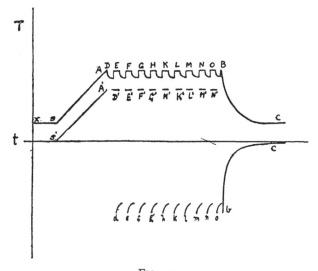

FIG, 11,

maximum of tension at A. But though the physical pain remained present until B, in imagination the child started to *think* of the bedclothes being put on long before this happened, and obtained very definite psychic pleasure from this imagination, by means of a series of psychic tension discharges at D, E, F, G, etc The pleasure obtained by these discharges is represented by the projected curves, d, e, f, g, etc., while intermittent consciousness of pain is shown by the short line, D', E', F', G', H', etc. His own description of this early stage was that of an alternating series of pain-pleasure feelings, in which, as weeks went by, the pleasure predominated more and more and the pain was less and less. And it is here that we begin to see the influence of habit at work, for from his own description of it, the constant repetition of this curious occupation made the obtaining of pleasure much easier. How much habit had to do with it will be seen when we examine the third stage of development in this case. After a few months he would find other thoughts beginning to intrude, and would temporarily forget about the *object* of the clothes being thrown off, would forget to keep his imagination fixed on the ultimate pleasure, but, nevertheless, he still remained conscious as he said of the " pleasure of being cold," *the relief which was to come remaining unconscious.* We must account for this by the imagination having now become an unconscious or habitual factor.

The term " unconscious " is used in so many ways psychologically, that I will pause here to limit my meaning very definitely. When I speak of a discharge of tension which was previously conscious having become unconscious, I merely indicate that by regular use a pathway or channel has been formed, by means of which that discharge can take place automatically without conscious direction. It may be that this is simply the result of special changes taking place in the synapses of various association nerve fibres in the brain —I do not know. We do know, however, that some such activity, as a result of habit, does become unconscious. The practised musician becomes unconscious of the exact fingering and thought by means of which he reproduces written music on the piano. The student is conscious of the meaning, but not of the spelling of words in front of him. The philosopher in the country may be quite unconscious that he is walking. A thousand oft-repeated habits become performed mechanically, through an established channel for the flow of energy, while the individual's mind is focussed consciously elsewhere. Therefore, when I refer to the imagination having become unconscious, I do not neces-

sarily mean that the imagination exists as
such at all, but that it has established a path
by means of habitual use, through which
tension can now be discharged without
conscious effort.   For the sake of continuity

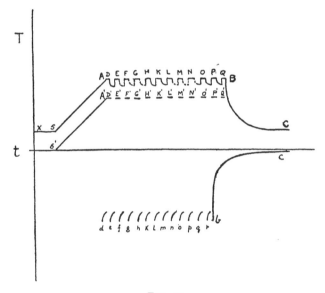

FIG. 12.

of thought and expression, however, I will
still continue to use the term, " unconscious
imagination."

Let us attempt to represent, in graphic
form, this third phase.   It will be of the same
nature as that shown in fig. 11, but we have

E

to represent at least some of the tension discharges as taking place unconsciously. This we can do in fig. 12, by using the dotted lines, D, E—G, H, etc., while by drawing a few of the lines heavily we represent occasions on which the discharge of tension becomes conscious. But since the *pleasure* attending the discharge was always conscious, the projected curves, d, e, f. g., etc., are none of them dotted, but remain as before.

We see, therefore, if we follow the actual happenings logically, and postulate an " unconscious imagination " carrying on the discharge of tension after a " habit path " has been established, that we may have an explanation of the apparent enjoyment of pain itself—of masochism—but we note that it is apparent only.

One other point which it is of the greatest importance to notice is, that the ideas which have in this instance ceased to be conscious, are those connected with the *anticipation* of the final act—his restoration of the blankets. That is to say, they are *ideas connected with fore-pleasure*.

We are now enabled to discover many similar cases to this in every-day life, and their mechanism will be clearer to us, though the history of them is not so clearly marked. We may compare it with the child who takes the tit-bit on its plate and puts it on one side, and saves it to the end of the meal. This, though trivial, is certainly a painful act in one sense ; that is to say, a state of tension is caused by denying oneself the immediate pleasure, but the imagination gives a definite discharge of this tension by means of the thought, " How pleasant it will be when I do eat it ! " Eating is deliberately postponed, and the tension due to a continual series of pain stimuli is discharged, which process we now call " *conscious fore-pleasure.*" This activity is in every way comparable with that shown in fig. 12.

I may add that the patient I have referred to showed other unusual forms of his habit of utilising fore-pleasure unconsciously ; he was a bad stammerer, and this took the form of not being able to speak when in an important situation. Frequently he could not ask for a railway ticket, or a number on the telephone. Analysis showed that this particular form of stammering was due, at least in part, to the unconscious pleasure in the idea that when he did speak and overcome the difficulty it would be extremely pleasant.

His fore-pleasure took other forms also. In his fantasy he imagined running away with ladies and undressing them. At that point he found that he remained, and postponed indefinitely any sexual act. He preferred to continue in the state of fore-pleasure, rather than to complete the act, and lose the pleasure. He was also inclined to clothes fetishism.

The stammer was obviously painful consciously, the phantasy we have mentioned was obviously a state of tension giving pain, though not physical pain. In other words, he had gradually come to cling to a state of tension with a conscious or unconscious imaginative discharge of it, rather than proceed actually to discharge that tension and obtain the normal pleasure which would have ensued therefrom.

PART II

UNCONSCIOUS TENSION.

§1

WE considered at an earlier stage of this enquiry (fig. 4) that every animal must exist in a state of tension, which was termed "normal tension." It is due in the first place to its organic existence and the physical and chemical processes which that existence implies, and in the second place to stimuli coming from the environment, together with its responses to these. Here already some degree of consciousness is introduced, and in human beings psychic tension of various different kinds must be present as a factor in the normal tension. As we should naturally expect, therefore, the state of "normal tension" is not simple at all, but is a complex condition consisting of many "tensions" fused in a certain whole. Remembering this, however, we may treat it for the purpose of illustration as though it were a simpler state than is actually the case.

Let us remember also that as a rule we are

not fully conscious of this tension, or of its causes. As a rule, normal tension, as well as many of the elements which make it up, never does reach consciousness at all.

It is obvious that it will be very difficult, if not impossible, to draw a boundary line between "normal" tension and that super-imposed by special stimuli, at any rate in beings possessing imagination and purpose; and we shall not attempt to do so here, but must keep as far as possible to more obvious aspects of the matter.

We have hitherto considered the question of pleasure which is obtained from the discharge of tension which is above the normal, *i.e.*, imposed by special stimuli. We have not considered whether the normal tension can in any way be relieved, nor what forms of pleasure can be obtained by so doing. We shall now, therefore, proceed to examine this problem.

There must be many forms of normal physical tension which it is hardly possible for us to suppose could wholly be relieved. There must be certain limits, for the life of the organism to continue, below which its physical tension does not fall, and above which it does not rise, and between which its states of tension fluctuate, and within which there is a narrower limit which we may think of as the normal, for the organism concerned. It is obvious that this will hardly be maintained as a constant, but will alter during the course of its existence, and may be subject to many modifications. Different individuals will also be likely to show a relatively higher or a lower normal level of tension maintained. The capacity for sustaining alterations of tension will certainly also vary in individuals.

Sleep is usually the condition of minimum tension ; at least this appears probable. But at most it represents only a reduction of tension. For instance, that caused by the presence of hydrogen-ion concentration in the blood, which leads to the act of respiration, must continue even during sleep, and there are many other sources of physical tension which similarly cannot be removed.

Yet many slight physical discomforts, of which we are not, when awake, fully conscious, as well as mild states of psychic tension which we might place in the same category, are relieved during sleep, and also by means of other methods which displace them further from consciousness.

We may refer once again to the infant ;

but let us first reconstruct our curve (fig. 13) of normal tension. As before, we will presume the pre-natal state to be one of a certain unknown tension, represented by the line X—S. Tension due to the act of birth must now be represented, by a sudden rise, S—A, followed by a fall, A—B—C.

At C the child is once more warm, peaceful

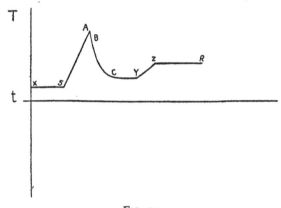

FIG. 13

and fed, but it is breathing and trying to adjust itself to the new environment in which it is existing. It is in the state which we call normal physical tension (normal, that is, to this period of its life), represented by the line, C—Y. Gradually, at a little later stage in this existence, it will start having interests and desires, fears and worries, some of which

are never again completely removed from it.
There is always the danger before it of something which it ought not to do, or of placing
itself in a position where pain may ensue.
With the rest of humanity, it has to be in a
condition of watchfulness, in one way or
another, and, with its developing consciousness, forms of tension which are thus purely
psychic are added to the psychic equivalent
of the previous physical tension, $e.g.$, the
increasing range of its sense experience, and
this is represented by a rise, Y—Z, until a
maximum normal tension, Z—R, is maintained, due to both physical and psychic
factors. I cannot represent all the elements
which will form part of this, nor its fluctua-
tions, nor the period of growth over which it
must be supposed to take place. This normal
tension will obviously vary enormously, as
we have already said, in different individuals,
not only in amount, but in stability, according
on the one hand to the sensitivity of the
individual, and on the other to the nature and
frequency of the stimuli imposed by environment. We may here observe the importance
of regulating normal tension in the infant.

Now we should suppose that there would be
a tendency to attempt continually to reduce

or discharge this tension ; and, indeed, that appears to be an underlying reaction throughout all life. It is as though this tension were accompanied by manifestations of pain or strain, usually unconscious—we only occasionally experience what we call a sense of tension—or, if the phraseology is preferred, it is as though manifestations of " pain " were continually trying to become conscious as a result of tension, whether normal or otherwise.

In point of fact, we do actually find both by observation of the infant and by psychological analysis of the adult, that this state of normal tension is one which we are constantly attempting to relieve, the continual partial releases of which, in successive activities and mental states, produce the mildly pleasurable tone of ordinary life.

But as we have seen, there are other more definite means of such relief. The infant spends most of its time in sleep, and thus retires to some extent from the state of tension, and from any effort to adapt itself to its environment, which causes that tension, slight though this effort may be. *And the infant will naturally automatically associate any of the causes which send it to sleep with this state of tension-relief.*

Thus, rocking the infant is a repetition of the movement experienced *in utero*, when the mother walked, and when it was in a state of sleep and minimal tension ; now rocking sends it to sleep. Similarly, warm clothing, after it has been cold or bathed, is a repetition of the condition of warmth *in utero*, and tends to send it to sleep. Again, feeding the infant also induces sleep in the same manner as it does in adults, and in many animals, possibly by a determination of the flow of blood to the viscera away from the brain. But in any case, whatever the cause, the result is the same, food certainly induces sleep, and after a meal the child naturally falls asleep, and will, therefore, form unconscious associations of food with reduction, not only of the specific hunger tension, but of normal tension also.

The sucking of the child is a special aspect of the matter and more complex. It satisfies a certain oral tension which we need not enter into here. We can see, however, that sucking is associated with feeding, and, therefore, in the first instance, by a similar association, it becomes related to sleep. We should expect that if these ideas be correct, at a later period of life, rocking or its substitute, warmth or its substitute, and sucking or feeding or its

substitute, would have, from unconscious
association and feeling, the effect of reducing
or compensating for the normal tension of the
individual after he has left his infantile life
behind.   I think we shall find this to be the
case.

We will take the example of sucking, for
we can follow this to a large extent through
life.   After the mother's breast the child
proceeds to suck an artificial teat, and in many
instances will not go to sleep without it.   It
appears to obtain a positive enjoyment from
it.   At a little later period it enjoys sucking
sweets, quite apart from whether it is hungry
or not, and these serve a two-fold purpose.
They not only give the pleasure of sucking,
but they give the child the sweet flavour which
may be associated with the flavour of the milk
at the mother's breast.   They probably have,
in fact we know them to have, other associations, but we are only concerned with the
development of one infantile habit.   Not only
does the child continue through a long period
of years to enjoy sucking sweets, but it will
form other habits of sucking, for instance,
smoking, sucking the end of a pen or pencil,
etc.   If, at the end of this chain of events, we
ask the individual : " What pleasure do you

get from smoking ? " he will very likely reply :
" I like it because it soothes my nerves."
That phrase tells us that just the same is
happening in adult life through the medium
of his cigarette as previously happened with
the dummy teat when sucked by the baby,
although when he is not soothing his " nerves "
by means of this cigarette, he is very likely
not conscious that he has any " nerves " at
all. The cigarette, however, by bringing in
its train all associated feelings right back to
those of sleep, is now giving him a form of
pleasure which is a reduction of normal
tension, and we see that the pleasure is, in
fact, a positive pleasure, that is, a pleasure
obtained where no conscious tension previously
existed. The same principle appears to hold
good, that is, that pleasure is only produced
as a result of relief of tension, and not in itself
by means of a pleasurable stimulus. This
is shown in fig. 14.

X—S represents a full state of normal
tension, including that produced both by
physical and psychic stimuli. From X to S
there is neither conscious pain nor pleasure
apparent, but at the point S the cigarette is
lighted, and the tension reduced by means
of the unconscious associations connecting

sucking with rest and sleep. At the point A the limit of reduction of tension is reached, and at C the cigarette is finished and tension increases again.

From S to C we speak of enjoying the cigarette, that is, we apparently have positive pleasure. This positive pleasure is apparently attained because the normal tension has been

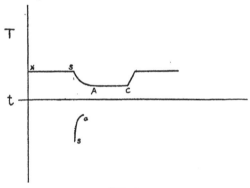

FIG. 14.

reduced each time the cigarette was sucked, but more especially, as introspection will again tell us, when it was first lighted. We ought, of course, to have represented this curve by a series of reductions as in fig. 11. But for simplicity we have merely represented one puff of the cigarette, and one experience of pleasure, s—a.

If, however, instead of a cigarette, we take

the example of alcohol, which, as has been recently stated by the Medical Research Committee, acts entirely as a narcotic on the higher centres, the truth of this statement is even more clearly seen.

The report states* : "We may notice at once that even under these conditions alcohol produces to some degree that effect which, perhaps more than any other, is the secret of its charm, its well-nigh universal attraction for the human race, namely, a sense of careless well-being or of bodily and mental comfort. In so far as this sense of well-being is of bodily origin, it is no doubt largely due to a flushing of the skin with blood that abolishes all sense of chill ; but it is due also in part to a blunting of the sensibility to the small aches and pains, and a thousand hardly distinguishable sense-impressions which, except in those in perfect health, contribute to tip up the balance of bodily feeling-tone to the negative, or un-pleasant side. In so far as this effect is primarily mental, it results from the blunting of those higher mental faculties which lead us to 'look before and after, and pine for what is not,' and harass us with care for the

* *Alcohol : Its Action on the Human Organism.* Second Edition, revised,

future and a too sensitive self-consciousness
for the present . . . the direct effect of alcohol
upon the nervous system is, in all stages, and
upon all parts of the system,* to depress or
suspend its functions ; that it is, in short,
from first to last a narcotic drug."

We see here why alcohol is so much more
effective than a cigarette in producing a
feeling of well-being, that is, in reducing the
state of normal tension.

It flushes the skin and makes it warm,
that is, it brings about the pre-natal condition
in this respect, or, at any rate, the infantile
condition. Secondly, whereas the action of
the cigarette was by means of its unconscious
associations with sucking—with possibly a
very slight physical narcotic effect—the
alcohol reduces the actual physical tension,
for, by its blunting the higher centres of the
brain, some of the stimuli are actually cut off
from consciousness. Thirdly, drinking (frequently sipping) is allied to sucking, so that
we get a combination of psychic associations
leading to reduction of tension, with actual
reduction of physical tension. If sufficient
alcohol is taken, the normal tension is almost

---

* For a possible exception to this statement in the case of the
nerve centres of respiration, see p. 75–76. *Op cit.*

entirely eliminated, as shown in fig. 15 by the line S—C, where each successive lowering of tension, L, M, N, O, represents a fresh dose of the drug. If sufficient be taken without its being rejected by the mechanism of the body, the tension will be altogether reduced at C, when death will ensue.

A rather different series of events may take

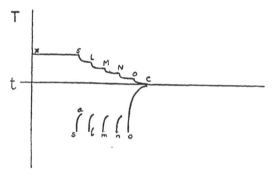

FIG. 15.

place with other drugs. Alcohol does not, in itself, act as an excitant. But for other reasons, when inhibition has been removed by alcohol, people may become excited. Certain drugs, however, act as stimuli, and cause an actual state of excitement due to their stimulating effect. But such drugs also have their action on the higher centres of the brain, or on certain parts of the body, in

F

reducing their susceptibility to pain and
worry.   Hence the stimuli which they impose
are less effective as pain producers than the
stimuli which they oppose, and we are still
correct in saying that the positive pleasure
obtained from such drugs is ultimately due
to the reduction of tension.   Now let us look
at some of the other examples suggested and
I think we shall see that they may be accounted
for in a similar way.

Let us examine the pleasure conferred by
the sunshine or sunrise.   Light itself is a
stimulus which, if it be bright enough, is
certainly of a definitely painful character.
We also know, however, that light is perceived
as the result of the higher wave lengths which,
in their lower form, produce the phenomenon
known as heat, and ideas of light and heat are
frequently interchangeable as associated ideas
in the mind.   When the sun shines, we feel
warm, and the primary pleasure that any
individual takes in manifestations of this
kind is in the feeling of warmth.   Now, in this
country at any rate, almost the first unpleasant
tension which the infant meets with is that
caused by cold, and warm clothing or warm
sunshine represents the reduction of that
cold-tension.   On the whole, throughout life,

the individual is having a struggle to keep his body in the proper condition of warmth, that is to say, he is always in a state of normal tension. The face, the hands, and the feet are, except on specially warm days, continually in a state of mild tension due to cold stimuli for, for the most part, the temperature of the atmosphere is less than the temperature of the body. This varies in different people and at different times, and we associate, to a large extent, feelings of chilliness with a cloudy sky and darkness, for at night it is colder than in the day. We speak of a fire *looking* cheerful, because we associate the ideas of light and warmth, and we see here one of the primary factors in the pleasure of alcohol, which flushes the skin, both of the hands and the face, and assists in obliterating the tension due to cold in these parts.

We know that, after a series of winter days, we welcome the sun first of all, not because of its beauty, but because of its warmth, but since we associate the light of the sun with the heat of the sun, just as we do the " cheerful " appearance of a fire with the heat of the fire, we are inclined to call it beautiful because it gives us pleasure by reducing our tension, and it is not a far cry to say that by a series

of associations all bright things will ultimately
tend to cause, in the imagination—consciously
at first and then unconsciously—the discharge
of what we term normal tension. So that we
may ultimately come to appreciate a sunrise
simply because it reduces the state of tension
which we are not fully consciously aware of
before.

For this reason some people take pleasure
in getting up to see the sun rise, for it brings
with it associations of warmth after the cold
night, of a fire on a cold day, or of clothing to
the cold infant. This is a psychic means of
reducing normal tension comparable with the
cigarette, or more strictly still, with the boy
who deliberately made himself cold in bed in
order to make himself warm again. The
stimuli in themselves are not pleasurable
stimuli, but are pleasurable because they
counteract other stimuli and so reduce the
condition of tension. From this we may
ultimately see that all forms of what may be
termed peaceful beauty—pictures, seascapes
and so forth—tend to cause us pleasure from
the fact that they actually do reduce the
normal tension.

This is, of course, quite apart from such
forms of beauty as we appreciate from the

sexual point of view. These act as stimuli to increase our state of tension, and their pleasure aspect belongs to the category of fore-pleasure, which we discussed in relation to the boy who threw off his bed-clothes, the pleasurable experience being that of the unconscious anticipation of the relief of sexual tension.

It is the same with a variety of stimuli, apparently pleasant in themselves. They will be found, either directly or by association of ideas, to produce a reduction of some form of tension. The question of why certain stimuli do normally act in this way, a sweet taste, or a combination of harmonious sounds, for instance, would lead to very difficult issues. Yet, in general, we know perfectly well that the state of tension of the individual, and not the stimulus, determines the pleasure or displeasure he feels at any event. If I wish to take up biology or to learn French, I am pleased when the opportunity is presented to me ; if I do not, the opportunity is indifferent to me, and I do not notice it ; on another occasion the suggestion might even annoy me. The same holds good of seeing the sun rise.

Let us look, for a moment, at an apparent exception. It is not uncommon, probably,

to hear someone say : " A cigarette helps to
concentrate my mind when I am tired," as
though the pleasure of smoking appeared
to raise, rather than relieve, tension. Here,
however, the fact of the matter is, that the
cigarette has relieved a sum of mild tensions,
among which the only one consciously perceived by the individual was that produced
by the toxic effect of a slight state of fatigue,
which were opposing some other aim which
required a different form of tension to attain
its end, and discharge the individual's psychic
energy satisfactorily. Hence the principle
still holds good.

We see then, that so far, most examples
will fit in with this hypothesis, and by means
of it even the apparent enjoyment of pain
can be accounted for, and the enjoyment of
the postponement of pleasure, and other
experiences of a similar nature, which are
difficult to account for without it. We shall
obtain further support of it, however, if we
carry our ideas a stage further.

It may be interesting to note here that we
can now divide pleasure into two fairly
distinct categories—on the one hand, peaceful
or calm pleasures, and on the other hand,
pleasures accompanied by excitement. The

peaceful or calm pleasures are apparently those associated, for the most part, with the reduction of normal tension, with the soothing feeling produced, not by reduction of abnormal tension, but by removing normal tension and approaching that supposed calm or peaceful condition of Nirvana, wherein there is assumed to be no tension. The pleasures accompanied by excitement are those obtained by imposing abnormal tension, which is then reduced. In the case of beings endowed with imagination, added stimuli are frequently deliberately sought, in order to produce abnormal tension, which they then reduce psychically or physically, or both.*   For instance, in a game of tennis, we produce a condition of tension in which we fear to miss a stroke or lose the game, and if this occurs, we have a moment of psychic pain, relieved by the next successful stroke that is made.   So that a game of tennis, or indeed any other game, is a continual alternation of production of tension and relief of it.

The same would apply to a game of poker and the fascination of gambling, wherein the possibility of loss causes a high state of psychic

* Very possibly the process of reducing abnormal tension also results in a more efficient reduction of the normal tension as well.

tension which, in the mind of the gambler, is amply compensated for by the pleasure of reducing that tension when he wins.

§2

We might, before proceeding to examine our hypothesis on other grounds and in other directions, again further examine the action of fore-pleasure in daily life.

If we consider the interest that a person takes in his work, we shall find that that same interest is in the nature of an unconscious discharge of tension. In the first place, the object of any work is to accomplish something, and the predominating interest is frequently in the final accomplishment, and not in the work itself. Thus many a man would like to possess a beautiful garden, but he would abhor making it, digging and planting, etc. And, in fact, he pays somebody else to do this part for him for that reason. On the other hand, one may be so constituted, that the actual making of the garden becomes in itself a pleasure. I have designed, and for the most part constructed with my own hands, a small rock garden. It is now finished, and there is no more room for working, and with the

finishing of it, I have lost all interest in it.
In the ordinary course of events, I dislike
digging in clay very much, and wheeling
barrows about, etc., but during the building
of this garden, I enjoyed every moment of the
work. What was happening was, that I was
anticipating completion unconsciously, and enjoying by a psychic discharge of tension what
would otherwise have been an unpleasant task.
We see that this is strictly comparable with
the example of the boy, who, throwing off
the bedclothes, enjoyed unconsciously the
situation when he was cold, and that the same
factors which cause masochism on the one
hand, when turned in a useful direction, tend
to make an individual efficient in the enjoyment of his labours. This, at a later period
we shall find to be of the utmost importance.

One very interesting and unexpected deduc-
tion seems as if it may follow from the
material we have so far been examining. We
have seen that apparently the primal instinct
in conscious animals appears, not so much to
be that of self-preservation, as that of avoiding
pain, and that, in order to do this, there
is a normal tendency to reduce tension
whenever it is caused, and even to get rid,
as far as possible, of that normal tension

which must always be present during life.
In order to do the latter efficiently, we
apparently attempt to get back to the state
that we were in before we were born, and,
in fact, such a state is approximated, of course,
by death, and unless some other factor were
at work we should be inclined to surmise that
one of our dominant instincts would be an
instinct to die rather than an instinct to live.

This rather startling idea, however, is not
so remarkable when we consider the factors
which actually stand between our possible
desires in this direction and our putting them
into practice.   In the primitive animal without
consciousness, death is prevented because it
is approached *via* the state of tension, from
which the animal automatically recedes
before it is high enough to bring death about.
And in the conscious animal the approach
to death is guarded on the one hand by pain,
produced by the actual physical tension which
would ultimately lead to death, and on the
other hand by anticipation, that is to say, by
psychic tension, due not only to the fact that
consciousness connects pain with death, but
that imagination also connects pain with the
unknown.   And even if we do not consciously
admit an existence after death, we uncon-

sciously recognise some possible unknown, which prevents us from voluntarily approaching this state of non-tension. But there is yet one other factor, perhaps the most important of all. It will be seen that in order to obtain pleasure, we have gradually accustomed ourselves to producing mild states of tension voluntarily, in order to discharge them again, and that amongst the various forms of pleasure which we take, *fore-pleasure, that is anticipation, both conscious and unconscious, is by far the most prominent.* Our greatest pleasure of to-day is the anticipation of the completion of that pleasure to-morrow (*e.g.,* interest in work), and if we contemplate death as to-morrow's portion for us, it means that we must *forego the fore-pleasure of to-day.* If the child is told that the toy will not be given to it to-morrow, it becomes unhappy now, having lost its fore-pleasure, and if the thirsty man is told that he will not receive a drink at the end of the journey his fore-pleasure of anticipation at once disappears, just as the boy who threw off his bed-clothes could obtain no pleasure if the bed-clothes were taken away from him altogether. Thus fore-pleasure acts as a main determinant which prevents us from discharging tension

by means of death, and we may deduce that
it is only when all fore-pleasure has been taken
away by some acute state of tension, either
physical or mental, or when a mind has been
so formed that fore-pleasure in the ordinary
affairs of life has not become a sufficiently
developed habit to carry the individual
forward, that any person will voluntarily seek
to reduce his tension completely. In such
cases, however, we should expect suicide to
result, as merely the fulfilment of the natural
instinct for death, or rather for a state of non-
tension, which is otherwise countered by the
various factors we have mentioned. Indeed,
I have in mind two recent patients who were
would-be suicides. One refrained on one
occasion as she wished to follow the hounds
the next morning and so postponed the
attempt till after this event. The other, a
young medical student, refrained as he was
ardently looking forward to a dance in three
weeks time. In both these cases other forms
of fore-pleasure had temporarily disappeared,
and only these remnants remained to guard
the gates of death.

This leads us on to a consideration of such
factors as hope and fear, and their place in the
hypothesis which we have discussed.

§3

We have already seen that the imagination can produce forms of tension and can also act as a means of discharging tension. And the latter we have already examined at some length.

It remains for us to consider in slightly more detail what part the imagination plays in producing tension. If a school-boy knows that in half-an-hour's time he is going to be caned, he reacts in many ways as though the caning were already there, and is psychically in a state of tension. He is informed that he is to appear before the headmaster in half-an-hour's time for the purpose of being caned. His tension, as the time of the thrashing approaches, becomes more acute. The actual thrashing takes place over a short period. Here we have an immediate access of anticipatory pain, which we call fear. It may be so great in some circumstances that the small boy will actually weep long before the thrashing takes place, and it is thus comparable with the state of pain produced by hunger, or by an actual thrashing which takes place without fore-warning.

We can now view the fear as *fore-pain, i.e.,*
anticipatory pain in imagination, in just the
same way as we view anticipatory pleasure
in the imagination as *fore-pleasure.* This leads
us on to enquiring whether, in connection
with pain, there is anything which is equivalent
to *unconsci us* fore-pleasure, which we found
to be one of the dominant forms of pleasure
which induced us to continue life. We
remember unconscious fore-pleasure was a
condition in which the end had been lost sight
of in consciousness, but a channel had been
formed through which a discharge of energy
took place, as a well-established habit. Let
us, therefore, look for such a state in connection with pain, *i.e.,* a state of high tension
the cause of which has been lost sight of in
consciousness, or has never been known, and
yet has a form of pain connected with it.

We do find something approaching this
condition in the phobias, and in some forms
of anxiety. In these conditions we find a
person developing a state of fear which he is
completely at a loss to give a reason for, or
he may have a fear placed on some objective
which his reason tells him is not appropriate
for fear. Indeed, although the cause of a
phobia is often unconscious, we know that a

very high state of tension is present in many
instances, and it is here that psycho-analysis
helps us, for we realise indeed that the cause
of fear has been lost sight of and that some
quite unsuitable object has been substituted.

In pursuing this matter into the idea of
anxiety, however, we meet with difficulties,
partly owing to the indefinite nature of our
definitions. For on the one hand the words
fear and anxiety are frequently used as though
they were interchangable terms, on the
other hand, there are various conditions in
reference to which the term anxiety is used,
which do not appear to be identical when
examined more closely. We may, however,
say that in anxiety there is a condition of
tension with a *degree of unconsciousness present.*
On the one hand the cause of the tension
may be unknown—on the other the cause
may be either only partially in consciousness
or the relief of tension uncertain of fulfilment.
" Hope " is very closely allied to anxiety, and
since the meaning of the term is not so
obscured, we can commence with a definition
of hope in terms of tension. Hope is a form
of fore-pleasure. We at once see that in hope,
the discharge of tension is not necessarily
unconscious, but is a possible, though doubtful,

consummation. Where the discharge of tension is certain, as in the case of the child who knows that it will be given a present in the course of two hours, we find definite fore-pleasure in possession. Where the discharge or tension is not certain, as in the case of the child who is uncertain whether it will obtain that pleasure, the imagination of that pleasure still forms fore-pleasure, but it is in conflict with the fear of not receiving the discharge of tension, and the conflict is manifested as anxiety and hope. We see that hope is constituted of two determinants. On the one hand is fear, which is repressed and partly unconscious (an unconscious fore-pain), and on the other is conscious fore-pleasure of which the outcome is uncertain.

In dealing with anxiety, we are also in difficulties, partly because physical symptoms are taken as entering into a syndrome, which is described by this term. I shall, therefore, do no more than indicate by one or two examples that in anxiety tension is present, but with a factor of uncertainty or uncon-sciousness concerning it. A simple case of anxiety is well exemplified in a runner before a race. The runner has definitely produced in himself a state of tension in the imagination for the purpose of relieving it by the pleasure produced when he is proclaimed the winner of the race. But immediately before the race, he will exhibit signs of mild anxiety. On the one hand, he is obtaining fore-pleasure in the thought that he will win the race, and, on the other hand, he is obtaining fore-pain by the thought that he will lose the race, and this conflict, because he is not considering it consciously all the time, and it is directed to an uncertain end (for he is not certain that he will win or lose the race), manifests itself in the form of anxiety.

Another example of anxiety is frequently seen in many so-called cases of shell-shock. The opposing forces are again those of fore-pain and fore-pleasure. The fore-pain of death or pain is present. The fore-pleasure of life and pleasure is present. The imagination first fixes upon one and then upon the other, but in neither case is there either *definite fore-pain*—for the man does not know that he will die—nor is there *definite fore-pleasure*, for the man does not know that he will live. There is thus a state of uncertainty —a lack of full consciousness of facts, which brings anxiety about as before.

The other cases to which the term anxiety is

G

applied, and in which general irritability, nervousness and physical disturbances are present, possess too many other determinants to treat them thus simply.   For instance, in the anxiety neuroses, we do not know definitely whether the mental tension causes the physical symptoms or *vice versa*, and it is not my intention at this early stage to cite any very complicated mechanism as example.   I shall, therefore, leave this subject of anxiety and hope, in what I fear is a very incomplete state, but one which will at least prove an indication of its position with regard to tension.

PART III

LOVE AND HATE

§1

As a final consideration in this preliminary thesis, we may suggest the allocation to their apparent positions, of the affects of love and hate, and we shall see once more that they apparently fall into line with the general hypothesis we have stated. If we take hate as representing all forms of dislike, whether great or small, we shall see that hate is that affect thrown on to the cause, or apparent cause, of any state of tension.

If we take such a primitive state of tension as the one which produces thirst, we shall see that our hatred is directed, not to thirst, but to the desert through which we happen to be travelling, which is the cause of that thirst, or to the sun's ferocity, which has dried up the water, and is therefore, ultimately, also the cause of thirst.

If we watch the apparent emotions of the lower animals, we observe at once that animals that are maltreated hate the person who maltreats them, just as boys who are regularly caned by a certain master, hate the master and the cane.

It is not at present necessary to pursue this question further, as apparently all dislike falls into this category. If we turn our attention now to love, using this word in its broadest sense, and including in it all forms of liking, we see that love is that affect which is directed towards any object which causes pleasure, that is, any object which relieves our tension ; from the love we possess towards the cigarette which relieves our normal tension, to the love we possess towards the water, the public-house, and the innkeeper, who conjointly relieve our thirst, and the love we possess towards our parents, who provide us with the food, raiment, and other necessities for relieving various other tensions of life.

Exactly the same also applies to the erotic love which ultimately relieves our sexual tension. We see here at once a curious thing, that since there can be no loss of tension without tension having first been produced, and also there can be no pleasure without pain or potential pain having first been present, so finally, it may be there can be no love unless hate or potential hate has first existed. At first sight this seems difficult to fit in with our usual ideas, but if we take two factors into consideration, I think the matter will become more obvious.   In the first place we find in the infant both love and hate are directed towards the same person alternately.   If we prefer to speak more colloquially, we can say " like and dislike." The infant who has gained no ideas of duty or other conventional standards by means of its environment, directs dislike towards that person who causes it to be cold by undressing it, or who interferes by punishment with its desires in any way, and even in such an apparently trivial matter as taking it away from the breast when it desires to suck, we find that it shows temper, and every sign of dislike towards the mother, in spite of the fact that it is simultaneously showing signs of love towards that part of the mother—namely, the breast—which it desires.

Or we may take an example from animal-life, which is quite commonly seen, namely that of the dog.   The dog which at most times will show every sign of love towards its master, will growl and bare its teeth when it sees the bath being prepared for it, or is threatened with a stick.   Indeed, in the former instance we can very readily see the extreme transition which takes place, for while it shows every sign of disliking the master before the bath, after its bath, when he is rubbing it down with a towel and making it comfortable again, it will bark and dance round him, with more pleasure than at normal times, and both in the case of the dog and in the case of the child, the giver of the pain has also been the giver of the pleasure, and hate has been followed by love.

There are other reasons, however, why this is not obvious in daily life, and why we are not conscious of hate towards most individuals in the same degree as we are conscious of our love.   In the first place, in the case of the child, for instance, the preponderating influ- ence is in favour of the mother, for she does not cause anything like as much tension as she removes.   Hunger, for instance, due to the tension of the child's stomach, is not ascribed to the mother, yet the mother gives the pleasure by reducing that tension.   Physical pain due to accidents is not caused by the mother, yet the mother soothes the child and again reduces the tension. Fatigue is not caused by the mother, but the mother rocks the infant to sleep, and reduces the tension. Hence, although love may not exist wthout hate, the hate may be largely unconscious and divided, and the love may very well predominate through being conscious and concentrated.

The second factor which comes into play is that our tendency is to prolong our pleasures —to keep the result of a continual discharge of tension in consciousness, while it has already been seen that there is an equal tendency to keep the tension itself away from consciousness. We live, for the most part, in a continuous unconscious discharge of tension which we have called fore-pleasure. For the same reason there will be a tendency for hate to be minimised and unconscious, for it belongs to the unpleasant, and for love to be prolonged and conscious, for it belongs to the pleasant, and, therefore, for love to occupy a predominant place in our lives, rather than hate.

Thirdly, our training and environment constantly suggest to us the duty of love and the abomination of hate, and this cause is, therefore, another determining factor, producing love in consciousness, and keeping hate in the background. There are, probably, other factors at work which it is, however, not necessary for us to go into in this general scheme, but it is necessary to point out one further thing—that just as pain appears to be proportional to the amount of tension, and pleasure to the rate of discharge of tension, so hate is likely to be proportional to the tension, and love to the rate of discharge of the tension. So that hate and love are not diametrically opposed, any more than acceleration and velocity are diametrically opposed. Hence, just as pleasure may be great or small, in any given instance, for a given height of tension, according to its rate of discharge rather than according to the amount of tension, so love may be great or small in a manner not proportional to the amount of hate first induced, and the two cannot be directly related to one another by saying that the more one hates the more one loves. For they are different affects following different laws.

PART IV

SUMMARY

LET me now summarise the essential axioms which stand out as a result of the hypotheses I have been considering :—

(1) In the conscious animal pain is the conscious affect accompanying tension, and it is proportional to the tension, but modified by the sensitivity of the cell or individual on the one hand, and by the kind of stimulus on the other hand.

(2) All tension tends to cause those affects which can be classified as painful, and all stimuli therefore tend to cause pain.

(3) Pleasure is that affect which results in the conscious animal as a result of the discharge or neutralisation of tension. It is not, however, proportional to the amount of tension as in the case of pain, but has a relation to the rate of discharge of tension modified by the sensitivity of the cell or individual on the one hand, and the type of stimulus on the other hand, together with other possible determinants. It has a relation to the formula :—

$$\pi = \frac{dT}{dt}$$

where pleasure is represented by π

(4) Pain and pleasure are thus not diametrically opposed, nor are they on the same plane. They

93

cannot be represented in terms of one another any more than velocity and acceleration can be so represented. Pain and pleasure can exist together simultaneously in the same individual, and these affects do not mutually efface one another.

(5) The discharge of tension, particularly in the psychic plane, habitually performed through some channel, tends to be performed unconsciously. Thus an unconscious cause of pleasure may be present producing conscious affect, and pleasure may be attributed to the tension itself, whereby pain, under certain circumstances, seems to be a source of pleasure.

(6) The essential interest in work and life is the discharge of tension through habitually formed channels, in which the goal, though lost sight of consciously, remains the unconscious source of pleasure. So that fore-pleasure and unconscious fore-pleasure thus constitute the interest in continuing life.

(7) There appears to be no evidence for an actual instinct of self-preservation as such, but only for an instinct to avoid tension and pain, which acts as a preservative to life.

(8) We are continually in a state of normal tension, the causes of which we have grown used to, and are therefore not for the most part conscious of, but we continually try to attain pleasure by means of discharge of this tension.

(9) It would appear that another important instinct is that whereby we attempt to reduce tension to the minimum, which is re-enforced by our desire to obtain pleasure through the medium of a discharge of tension, and which would, were it not for the continual fore-pleasure, lead us inevitably to death, could that be attained without tension and pain.

(10) Pleasure may be divided into two categories: firstly, that attained by the discharge of normal tension, *i.e.*, tension unaccompanied by pain may be described as " calm " pleasure; and secondly, that attained by the discharge of tension, caused by added stimuli, which may be called "exciting" pleasure.

(11) Just as fore-pleasure exists, so does fore-pain. Conscious fore-pain, that is the anticipation of tension in the imagination, is termed fear. Where the fore-pleasure is an uncertainty, that is, where it is not known whether the thing will be consummated or not, and, therefore, where some sort of fear is present, two conditions may arise, on the one hand hope, and on the other anxiety. Both these conditions are due to a conflict between fore-pleasure and fore-pain, which may be partially unconscious or completely so.

(12) Hate is an affect directed towards any cause of tension. Love is an affect directed towards any cause of the relief of tension. Like pain and pleasure, these two affects may be present simultaneously, and though hate is likely to be directly proportional to the tension, modified by the sensitivity of the subject, love is not necessarily proportional to the amount of hate induced, but since it is dependent on pleasure, is likely to be proportional to the rate of discharge of tension, modified by those same variants which come into play in the case of pleasure.

PART V

Freud's Theory and the Present Hypothesis

§1

It will be of some interest to consider how far the hypothesis agrees with psycho-analytical theory in the examples cited. It will be remembered that Freudian theory connects Masochism, through its relation to Sadism, with Anal-erotism. In our explanation of Masochism as a prolongation of fore-pleasure in which, though pain is apparently enjoyed the pleasure is really taken in an unconscious anticipation of the relief of tension, we actually mentioned no anal element. There was, however, in the case cited, such an element present as an earlier manifestation of postponement. The details may be given.

My patient recollected that in early childhood he had been afflicted with what he considered was probably inflamation of the bowels. His memory concerning the illness was vague. He was, nevertheless, quite clear that as a result of this he was very much troubled with constipation in early childhood.

He was constantly given enemas by his mother, and almost daily she insisted on steaming his excretory organs by setting him on a utensil which contained nearly boiling water. Whilst he had a quite vivid series of pictures in his mind, he did not remember a single occasion on which any result had ensued ; but he had a strong belief that he generally delayed results, and the idea of delay at the present time gave him a sense of pleasure. If his present feelings and belief, *viz.*, that the end somehow caused pleasure, may be included, this may be taken as an example in which he had succeeded in obliterating end-pleasure from consciousness and perpetuating fore-pleasure.

He remembered with considerable accuracy a slightly later development of this. At this time (after the age of five) he did have a daily evacuation of the bowels, which he both dreaded and liked. He dreaded this only when constipated, but recalled pleasure in both the idea and the physical feeling of passing fæces immediately after the first acute pain had passed. On the whole, however, painful constipation was not very frequent, and the pleasure very much outweighed the pain.

We now come to an unusual form of activity of his mind during this period. He stated that he found the greatest pleasure of all to consist in calling to mind that he would not have to repeat the operation for another twenty-four hours. It is not quite clear whether this desire to postpone grew out of fear of pain or the desire of pleasure, and for that reason I did not include it in the earlier chapter of this work. He would consciously say to himself that he was free for twenty-four hours, and he would try to imagine from time to time as the day went on that there were still twenty-four hours of freedom before him. Significance attaches to this as showing the development of his pleasure in postponement, for on very many occasions he did not actually postpone his evacuation of the bowels, but would deliberately attempt evacuation unnecessarily, in order to have the pleasure of contemplating the idea that he would have another twenty-four hours' freedom. Whether in this case, as seems likely, the pleasure of postponement first arose from the postponement of pain, we cannot say ; but at any rate, quite apart from this, we see that the development of the Masochistic idea is in this instance in harmony with the theory that Masochism is of an anal origin.   It is, of course, possible, on the one hand, that in this case there was a still more remote origin, in which the anal incidents were but later grafts.   On the other hand it is equally possible that in other cases postponement of either pain or pleasure might take place at some other somatic level without passing through an anal stage ; but for the time we must leave the matter there.

§2

Let us now turn to another aspect of the question.   My theory of pleasure and pain, viz., that pleasure bears a relationship to the rate of reduction of tension due to stimuli, which tension tends to be represented in consciousness as pain, appears to be in close correspondence with certain expressions of Freud and others.*   On page 3 of Freud's *Beyond the Pleasure Principle*, occurs the hypothesis " that there is an attempt on the part of the psychic apparatus to keep the quantity of excitation present as low as possible, or, at least, constant," whence it follows that " all that tends to increase it must be felt as contrary to function, that is to say, painful."

* *Cf.* E. Jones, *Papers on Psycho-analysis*, p. 21.

He says on the preceding page that for the purpose of psycho-analytical theory, pleasure and pain can be considered "in relation to the quantity of excitation present in the psychic life, along such lines that pain corresponds with an increase, and pleasure with a decrease in this quantity," although he would admit no simple relationship between the strength of the feelings and the corresponding changes, least of all, a direct proportion between them. " *Probably*," he continues, " *the amount of diminution or increase in a given time is the decisive factor for feeling.* Possibly," he adds, " there is room here for experimental work . . ."

This is a proposition akin to that which I have sought to elaborate by synthetic and introspective methods, so as to carry our theory of feeling a few steps further than the position it appears to be in at present. Let us observe once *more*, that the pleasure-process represented by my hypothesis (fig. 3) is not a simple correlate of the curve representing reduction of pain, but has quite other factors. In no way is pleasure a simple antithesis of pain.

Again we find (page 71) the following : " The ruling tendency of psychic life, perhaps

H

of nerve life altogether, is the struggle for reduction, keeping at a constant level, or removal of the inner stimulus tension," a tendency which he seems to regard as at the root of the pleasure principle itself, which is described (page 81) as subserving the function of "rendering the psychic apparatus as a whole, free from any excitation, or (keeping) the amount of excitation as low as possible. We cannot yet decide with certainty for either of these conceptions." It follows that the pleasure principle, thus understood, is consistent with his so-called "death-instinct," *i.e.*, "partaking of the most universal tendency of all living matter, to return to the peace of the inorganic world "—" the reinstatement of lifelessness" (page 54). This itself, let us remember, is only a relative "peace." The correspondence between these passages and my thesis that every substance in a state of tension tends to reduce that tension is a close one, though I have striven through a different formula to reach the conception of this law, as I think it is, of a return to a state of non-tension. This, however, it is impossible in reality to reach ; only reduced tension, or a change of its mode, being ever attained. Freud has called this "universal tendency,"

I think, the "death-instinct." But even
death, which appears to our ordinary thinking
to possess quite a definite and fixed meaning, is
according to the line of thought here suggested,
an instinct, if such it may be called, per-
vading inorganic as well as organic matter,
which leads it to retire altogether from
material being. Every material substance
is in a state of tension, and as a result it is
continuously wasting and breaking up, and
according to the latest theories, ceasing to
exist as such. As Sir Oliver Lodge has
stated, there is only one thing known that
does not appear to undergo disintegration,
and that is the ether itself.

Yet neither of Freud's ideas that the
operation of the pleasure-principle is to keep
the psychic apparatus as a whole "free"
from any excitation, or to keep the excitation
"as low as possible," seems to account for
the class of reactions which are yet well within
the scope of operation of the pleasure-
principle, which consists in attaining an
actual temporary increase of tension by
added stimuli, in order *to secure increased
pleasure by its discharge*; a class of tension-
discharges which I have called the "exciting"

pleasures, in distinction to the "calm" pleasures which I have regarded as attributable to successive discharges of normal tension. In my view the living organism welcomes the majority of stimuli purely for the purpose of discharging tension and gaining pleasure quite apart from any previous stimulus.. Thus Freud's idea is that the organism welcomes stimuli in order to maintain itself in a state of rest, whereas mine is that it deliberately disturbs rest in order to obtain pleasure, although the attainment of pleasure, it is true, does bring it back to rest.

We have little indication in what this psychic tension actually consists, it is true.* Freud, when he says that excitation of certain instincts (those called speculatively the "life-instincts"), "bring with them states of tension, the resolution of which is experienced as pleasure," seems to regard this tension in consciousness as a distinct state thereof, which may be pleasant or unpleasant in itself. This appears to me misleading, and I am convinced that the issue will be clearer if we can regard the state of tension itself and its discharge as

* Cf. Op. cit. p. 35 : " The indefinite nature of all the discussions that we term metapsychological, comes from the fact that we know nothing about the nature of the excitation process in the elements of the psychic systems, and do not feel justified in making any assumption about it."

an integral part of the feeling-process, instead of as a separately apprehended state of consciousness.

What is needed now is a closer and more detailed analysis of the elements constituting what I have called normal tension, as well as the nature of this tension in application to mental processes : for the present this question has to be left as we must also leave that of the nature of the energy itself.

§3

Let us now turn to the question of how our hypothesis is related to the theory of the libido. Here we may be inclined to surmise that this theory will come later on to be in some respects differently stated. When we considered the most primitive acts of reproduction and of feeding, we saw no reason to consider either of them caused by anything but local states of tension. Coming to the higher animals, a similar series of facts is present. In the multi-cellular animals we find that local tension is conducted from one cell to another by means of simple protoplasmic processes or by nerve fibres, so that we get in the higher animals somatic tension conducted from one segment to another, either directly, or *via* the brain and spinal cord. In conscious beings this may be accompanied by feeling changes that are related to this tension.

Some segments may be more readily excitable than others, or be excitable in special ways, as those of the special sense-organs, in response to stimuli outside the organism, while other groups, like those of digestion or sex are particularly liable to be excited by stimuli arising both within and without the organism, and may be supposed the more readily and massively to transfer their tension to remoter parts of the organism.

In connection with this class of excitation, however, we introduce a factor which we term " instinct." That is to say we have introduced a new and unknown factor to account for the phenomena. Consciousness does not as a rule, present to us directly sensations or ideas of varying " tension," but presentations of objects and other purely mental images, with desires and aims in connection with these. But the states of tension are there persistently, whether they are consciously recognised as present or not.

The libido-theory is bound up with such a

theory of instinct, and the libido is assumed
to be the energy-charge of certain instincts.

The libido-theory proceeds on the basis of
assuming the sexual and other instincts as a
starting point, because this corresponds to the
data of our experience, and also because it has
been found by psycho-analysis that the tension
of this psycho-physical system (the sexual one)
is capable of very wide ramifications. Because
certain tensions are found to be specifically
sexual, certain other forms of local tension
participating in these states are themselves
taken to be fundamentally sexual. It has
been found in practice, for instance, that
psycho-neuroses yield to treatment based on
this theory when properly applied. In other
words, it is a theory that " works." It must
be conceded that practical investigation must
start somewhere, and there is no harm in
assuming " instincts." We are organic beings,
and we think organically as long as we possibly
can, in terms of the organism and its functions,
and in no sphere are we more inevitably
prone to do so than in the domain of
psychology.

Because in the adult, after the primary sex
organs have been educated, the remoter parts
of the body participate in the tension, it seems

far from necessary to assume that local tension in these remoter parts is originally, or even in infancy, of the same nature. Thus, while it is admitted that oral tension in late childhood or adult life may be of an erotic nature, it seems unnecessary to assume that the same is the case in very early infancy. Analysis does inevitably produce erotic associations to oral tension, since education and environment have conduced to bring the two together through the physical senses, or through association of ideas later developed. The mother, possessing the association already, will produce in the baby such habit-associations between oral stimuli and erotic tension by *e.g.*, frequently kissing it and encouraging it to kiss, or kissing other persons in its presence. Or she will similarly produce or strengthen other added series of associations between its mouth and anus by frequent giving of medicines *via* the mouth with the avowed purpose of producing defecation *via* the anus and so on.

Freud compares the sucking of the infant, the flushing of its skin, and final satiety in sleep, with the similar conditions attained after a sexual orgasm, and refers both of these to sexuality, though in the very young infant the material has not been mentally associated at all, nor has the local genital segment been associated through tension discharge with the local oral segment.

I am, of course, aware that the reference of the two conditions to sexuality does not rest only on the observed resemblance. That there is a resemblance is obvious, and that associations dating back to early childhood are bound to lead in the same direction is equally obvious, for environment has always inculcated these associations.

We shall, however, notice that the condition attained by the infant, and also at the end of sexual orgasm, are both equally explained by the other hypothesis. It will be remembered that the significance of the associations formed as a result of the earliest experiences of infancy between feeding, sucking and sleep (reduction of tension), were gone into in an earlier section of this book, and bear this out. We are always in a state of normal tension after birth, and are for ever endeavouring to escape that tension and return to the pre-birth condition, as simulated in sleep (reduction of tension), and we see the explanation herein. After the reduction of sexual tension the same happens.

It is not my purpose to go into this matter here ; indeed, it would be impossible to do so

on the evidence I have presented. Perhaps
it will be said that I have not adequately
stated the Freudian position as to this so-
called sexual manifestation in infancy. Or
it may be asked why these activities do
regularly reduce tension in apparently similar
ways ; or why the cultural environment does
regularly concur to transmit the same associations ; to all which the answer given will
bring us back in a circle to the instinctual
starting-point. This resembles the old riddle
as to the priority of the hen or the egg.

We must own that it cannot yet be said
certainly how far these and other forms of
tension-discharge familiar to us at present
may be innate, and how far really produced
by cultural associations, *vide* the useful
example with regard to " inherited " fear
reactions quoted from B. Kidd's observations
with the wild duck.

Because in one portion of the vast curve of
evolution our psychic manifestations participate in the sexual tension to a greater extent
than we were wont to think (so that the
libido-theory, as it stands at present, serves
to account for a great many of the observed
facts), we need not suppose that the energy
underlying these manifestations is necessarily

sexual. This is like attempting to judge the whole curve from too small a section of it before we have seen enough of it to be certain whether we are even dealing with a closed or an open curve.

It does not follow that the energy we study in sexual manifestations is ultimately " sexual" at all. To recognise this is not to disregard the truth in the observations that have been made on this section of the curve ; still less is it to disregard the very forceful reasons and the evidence which caused Freud to insist through all criticism and misunderstanding upon the so-called " libidinous " or sexual element of these manifestations. It was necessary to do so, yet it may be only part of the truth. Freud does not deny the possibility of other instincts than libidinous ones. He says, in the work I have often referred to here, that psycho-analysis has not yet enabled us clearly to demonstrate any others—which is a very different thing.

This is why I have suggested that the energy of the libido may be considered as emanating from any form of somatic discharge of tension, which may be only designated as sexual when it flows through sexual channels, i.e., involves the excitation of sexual segments

That under modern conditions we do actually find a sexual basis for a very large proportion of our activities, including the sublimated or non-sexual ones, is true, but this may very well be due to the fact that environment from infancy has repeatedly so directed our series of tension-discharges. It seems equally possible that with a different environment the same sublimated activities, or, indeed, more valuable ones might be arrived at by other channels ; and hence it seems equally possible that even now in some individuals such may be the case, and this may account for the fact that we frequently find during analysis, a difficulty in tracing some activity or characteristic which appears as though it ought to be simple, when we consider other factors in the same individual.

§4

The final point, which I should like to return to in conclusion, is the surmise of Freud in his intensely interesting speculative work *Beyond the Pleasure Principle,* as to the existence of a death-instinct, whereby he characterises a tendency to the reinstatement of an earlier condition.

The difference between this and my hypothesis appears to be that in my view this tendency is to escape tension, which would be equally well served by death or unconsciousness. Although death may be the result of the tendency, the supposed instinct is purely to escape tension.* In the same way there may be no need to postulate a life-instinct. In creatures possessing consciousness and imagination, at any rate, the instinct appears to be to prolong pleasure, and in itself this is again concerned with the management and discharge of tension in order to secure an adequate succession of such discharges. Its result is the apparent maintenance of tension and the prolongation of life. It leads to the introduction of new and complex phenomena, such as the postponement of immediate pleasurable discharge and the voluntary acceptance of pain in the hope of an ultimate discharge, factors which have had most important cultural results. Thus, we see how the pleasure principle also serves this so-called life-instinct, though it should not be called a life-instinct, except as a descriptive term,

---

* See also pp. 78 *et seq. supra.* The surmise regarding an instinct to die was introduced into my preliminary lectures some two years ago, when I was unaware of Dr. Freud's speculations on the subject in his work, *Beyond the Pleasure Principle.*

for in itself it is merely concerned with the economy of tension, although life may be prolonged as a result.

Ultimately, there may be but one tendency : as *instinct* it is at times difficult to view it, for it is possessed by inanimate matter as well as by living organisms.   This may be summed up in the former words of the author, " that every substance in a state of tension tends to reduce that tension."   But even in the most primitive animals the haven of non-tension is guarded by a gate of super-tension.   This cannot be ascribed to instinct, for it is ultimately physical, as far as we can see, and the cause of this peculiar arrangement is as yet veiled from us.